Reviews & Praise

"Karla's devotion and loyalty are immeasurable. Her own story of redemption frames the core of her belief system and fuels her endless passion for God and people. This book is like an alarm clock going off in the depths of your soul saying *TIME TO WAKE UP and TAKE CONTROL OF YOUR LIFE*. Karla makes the thread of God's grace through mind, body, and spirit so evident and beautifully weaves it through every facet of each chapter. Don't let fear hold you back from what God has in store for you. I am confident that *Divinely Fit* will break generational chains for many." *Rocio Castro-Robinson, VP of Marketing, Branding, & Licensing at ED Ellen DeGeneres and CEO of RDC Brand Consulting.*

"Karla shares her personal experiences and journey of faith with great vulnerability. By God's grace, she lives out the spirit, mind, body strategy powerfully. She has a genuine desire to encourage and help others and it shows." *Bonnie Solberg-Friend, Pastor's Wife and Former Women's Ministry Director*

"I was born a girl with pure thoughts, actions, and feelings. As I traveled through this journey into womanhood I (like many) have been exposed to unpleasant experiences, which brought on bad thoughts and bad habits. As a woman I have found myself on many occasions fighting against those bad habits and experiences. At times, to the point of exhaustion. I have said to myself "If I could do this all over again, it would be different." Divinely Fit spoke to my soul. As we all know we get ONE shot at life. I have come to understand that "Rebirth" does not take place through a blind leap of faith but through gradual changes. An ongoing process involving our Mind, Body, and most importantly our Spirit as encompassed in this book. It's time to overcome those fears and bad habits that only lead into temptation. It's time to be Divinely Fit! Thank you, for sharing you with the world KM. We love you." *Omayra Martinez-Baidy, Sudor Taino Instructor and Hartford Police Detective*

"Karla is an inspiring leader and instructor, but I never knew the difficulties she had to overcome. Wow! When she added the exercises at the end of the chapters, she's given you ways to put the concepts into *action*. It is a riveting read, very well written, with a recipe for action!" *John Kapral, Associate Accountant, Capital Community College*

"We all have our own stories of incredibly challenging situations, unique, yet so very similar to the personal ones shared in this book. Karla helps us to move forward in all our brokenness, suggesting ways to alter our perception of those situations. She gives us tangible ways to process all that hurt and insecurity, ultimately strengthening and freeing us to live passionately and transforming us into who God meant us to be. What an inspiring and Divine journey of healing so incredibly important for such a time as this!" *Carol Gingras, WEFC Community Group Member*

"Karla's message is one of faith, strength, and passion. Faith, in God and oneself. Strength, to overcome any obstacles. Passion, to help others achieve their goals." *Gary, Deputy U.S. Marshal, Retired*

"I am still trying to gage if women, girls, men, and boys are immune when they hear another person was molested in today's climate. Perhaps, the dog whistle will only be heard by those who can empathize first hand. As long as SHEROs like Karla continue to serve our community, be a voice for the vulnerable, and mentor for all of us, the whistle may turn to a megaphone, so everyone can hear." *Maria Furlow, Host & Executive Producer of Gyrl Sense*

"Karla uses a simple and sensible approach when speaking her life's truth. Her stories shared descriptively and with candor, are thought-provoking. With each chapter, the reader is drawn to each message and understands that in order to achieve balance in one's life, the relationship with your spirit, body, and mind must recognize God at its core and at its essence. Karla's words teach us what it means to be divinely fit." *Rossella Hara, 7th grade Language Arts teacher & Avid member of Sudor Taino Group Fitness*

"A perfect example of having true faith that guides you through all obstacles that life gives you. This book places that concept of hope and faith first which makes all things possible." *Debra A. Callahan, Auto Repair Shop Manager & Sudor Taino Member*

WISDOM & INSIGHTS SERIES

DIVINELY FIT

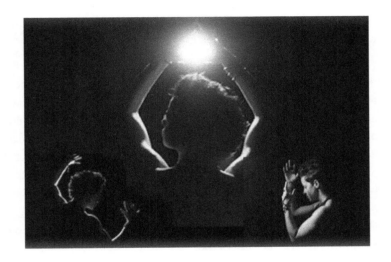

*A Spirit, Mind, Body Journey of
Struggle & Promise*

Karla Medina

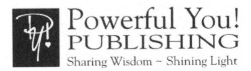
Powerful You!
PUBLISHING
Sharing Wisdom ~ Shining Light

DIVINELY FIT
A Spirit, Mind, Body Journey of Struggle & Promise

Copyright © 2018

The author of this book does not dispense medical advice or prescribe the use of any technique as a form of treatment for physical, emotional, or medical problems without the advice of a physician, either directly or indirectly. Nor is this book intended to provide personalized legal, accounting, financial, or investment advice. Readers are encouraged to seek the counsel of competent professionals with regards to such matters. The intent of the author is to provide general information to individuals who are taking positive steps in their lives for emotional and spiritual well-being. If you use any of the information in this book for yourself, which is your constitutional right, the author and the publisher assume no responsibility for your actions.

.

Published by: Powerful You! Inc. USA
powerfulyoupublishing.com

Library of Congress Control Number: 2018933554

Karla Medina – First Edition

ISBN: 978-0-9970661-8-0

First Edition March 2018

Body, Mind & Spirit: Inspiration & Personal Growth

Dedication

This book is dedicated to all those out there who believe they are "broken." May it help you understand that with God you can recover from any trauma and not only survive, but thrive. No matter what you have been through, you can be remade in the spirit and become divinely fit.

I also dedicate this book to the future generations; that as they walk through this world they may know the love, protection, and guidance of the Creator.

A special dedication to the resilient Taino Tribe, who cultivated La Isla de Puerto Rico, and to the survivors of Hurricane Maria who continue to cultivate the land today. A heartfelt dedication to the Sudor Taino tribe for allowing me to create a blessed space where members receive the love and support they need to explore their personal cultivation.

Most importantly, I dedicate this book to the collective, global effort to uplift, inspire, and heal the spiritual poverty of humanity.

Los amo a todos!

Table of Contents

Introduction

Over the years, I have collected stories, tips, mantras, quotes, teachings, and readings that address all manner of life challenges, yet in the end, they have all pointed me to the same advice template: Spirit, Mind, and Body. This sturdy, structured template can get you through any problem, whether it's at home or at work. It can even get you through a workout. Being physically and mentally fit, it seems, is incumbent on your spiritual fitness. On this I speak from experience. Every time I do not want to get up, get things done, eat right, get a workout in, or endure family or work problems, I need only call on the one thing I know won't fail me: the Divine, or GOD.

I certainly called on God many times while writing this book—in fact, I did so every time the doubts popped into my mind and began playing on a loop. Things like, "You can't write a book—you're not an expert on any particular subject matter," or "You don't know enough about life or the Holy Bible to give advice to others." With God, however, I realized that it is my very imperfection that lends me credence. You see, like all of you, I am imperfectly perfected, an everyday warrior. My life's journey bears this out: I was raised in the projects, in a single-parent household. I experienced child abuse and lost family and friends to gang violence and drug abuse; I've suffered from an eating disorder, loneliness, depression, fear, anxiety, and serious health issues; I've dealt with divorce, family battles, and more. In retrospect, I am grateful for those experiences, for without them I would not have found my spirit's divine direction. I would not have understood that God was always there; I just wasn't with God. So you see, I am not sitting on a pedestal, but down in the daily struggle, trying to achieve and maintain balance in all areas of my life. As I do this, my spirituality continues to evolve, helping me decipher what works for me. And in this complicated and challenging world, that is the best any of us can do.

This book is meant to comfort you, make you acknowledge your discomfort, and use it to be the best person that you can be. It is meant to give you a different perspective on your life and shift your focus toward creating transparency among your spirit, mind, and body. All too often we compartmentalize these areas—we think if we go to the gym three days a week to train our bodies and feed our Spirits at church on Sundays, we're doing our best. But if this is so, why are we still struggling with our weight, finances, and relationships? Oftentimes it's because we're out of balance—we've given our mind, with all its tendencies to overanalyze and criticize—the reins. I learned this lesson after years of daily struggle to balance life. Though I had achieved a lot, this struggle was exhausting. There had to be another way. In my search for deeper understanding, I realized that if my spirit was not right, then my mind and body certainly did not have a chance. (Though I had always believed in God, I began for the first time to truly exercise my spirit, and to create a "transparent bridge" between it and my mind and body). Using this spirit-mind-body template I noticed that I was growing stronger, experiencing shorter recovery times within life challenges, and inevitably becoming divinely fit. My wish for you is not that you follow my specific regimen, but that you use the lessons within to find what works for you.

That said, I'd like to explain my thought process while writing the book and offer some advice on how you can best utilize it. Essentially, it teaches you how to live less in the flesh and more in the spirit. As a follower of Christ and a proud member of God's army, I have often found myself trying to reconcile the Creator with His creation. While there are many beautiful things about our world, it is also fast-paced, complicated, and tumultuous, and I have often found myself overwhelmed by it. I have come to realize, however, that these times are opportunities to turn my focus to love. When your spirit is grounded in love, you remember to depend on your personal connection to God rather than what you perceive with your human eyes and mind. The troubles of the flesh lessen and often fall away, and you begin to walk through each day surrounded by an invisible safety net ensuring that you are never alone. Your love for God will spill over onto yourself and others around you. Whether you are a follower of Christ or not, if you rely on God (or Creator, Source, All That Is, etc.) He will help you break the chains and cycles of self-limiting beliefs holding you back and serve as a foundation for your journey to becoming divinely fit.

It is important to me that you understand why I chose to use Biblical quotes to illustrate the lessons in this book. First, the Holy Bible's proven factual and historical content makes it an unimpeachable source upon which I rely heavily on in my own life. Second, the sheer scope of the Bible means it lends guidance in virtually every situation and area of our lives. Third, the Bible provides constant reminders that despite our shortcomings, God's forgiveness and love for us knows no bounds. Lastly, it provides assurance that when we are weak in the flesh He will always guide us in the spirit. The Bible has inspired me—both in life and while writing this book—to focus not on the "*I can't*" (we have enough of that in our heads), but on the "He can!" As you read this book, you might find yourself turning to the Bible to expand upon the concepts.

You may also turn to other sources for guidance, though I challenge you to find one that offers all that the Bible does. The choice is yours. All I ask is that instead of spending your time trying to prove me or my references wrong, you spend it learning about the powerful spirit that lives within you.

This book is not just theoretical, but a practical, easy-to-follow strategy designed to rewire and realign the spirit, mind, and body. Each chapter focuses on a specific lesson—some will help you find and remove the "dark roots" of your anger, hurt, envy, or bitterness, and others will help you realize the truth and promise of God's Divine Light that moves in and around us. The lessons may be read sequentially or as needed to address a particular challenge you're facing. To this end, I have concluded each chapter with three simple exercises. The spirit exercises activate your connection to God and to the Higher Self within you. The mind exercises ask you to delve into the challenging aspects of your life, even those lurking deep below the surface, and bring them to the light. The physical exercises will integrate the spiritual message while igniting your body's feel-good hormones. All of the exercises are geared to promote an overall state of well-being that will take you through your day, each day, for the rest of your life.

Now, it's time for your spirit to emerge, "get right", and embrace the abundant blessings God has for you! It's time for you to *consciously choose* to embark on the journey to becoming divinely fit!

Namaste`,
Karla

The Struggles

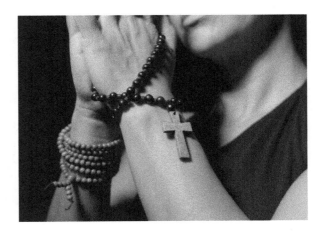

Everyone struggles with negative emotions like
bitterness, envy, and judgment;
they are part of the human condition.
The following chapters define those "dark roots" and
remind us that each day we are gifted with the choice to
acknowledge and excavate them from our lives.

The Struggle with Balance

Don't drink too much wine and get drunk;
don't eat too much food and get fat.
Drunks and gluttons will end up in a stupor
and dressed in rags.
Proverbs 23:20-21

We usually associate overindulgence with something that is bad for us—we eat too many desserts over the holidays or have a few too many cocktails on Friday nights. We don't realize that overindulgence is not about the particular behavior, but a lack of balance—meaning we can also overindulge in something that is generally considered healthy! In the days leading up to my first wedding, I developed an over-the- top-obsession with exercise. My desire to look the best and be the best drove me to work out at least a couple of hours each day, seven days a week! I even experimented with weight loss supplements and engaged in other practices that could have led to a full-fledged eating disorder. This was nothing new to me—I had been bulimic back in high school, while serving as captain of the cheerleading team. There was pressure to be "perfect," and bulimia seemed to work for some of my fellow cheerleaders. Sure enough, it did get me from a size 8 to a size 2! Unfortunately, I also became too frail to continue cheering. I clearly remembered the pitfalls of such an unhealthy obsession, yet there I was, pre-wedding (and later, post-pregnancy), thinking such behavior was the solution to my body image problems. Thankfully, my mind and body were abruptly halted by my spirit.

I have learned over the years that within the patterns and personal cycles we adopt, too much of anything eventually has its side effects. Though challenging at times, learning how to moderate everything on your plate will lead to success. Now, I am not talking about an actual plate of food; I am talking about your *life's plate*. I am talking about all the clothes you have in your closet with the tags still on them, the over-the-top Facebook posts, your constant complaining, indirect gossiping, undercover bragging, obsessively weighing yourself and working out, constantly comparing yourself to others, the different foods you eat depending on whether people are watching or not watching you, et cetera. Balance and moderation are rooted in spirit and hold the keys to healthy relationships with God, yourself, family, friends, food, exercise, shopping, and so on.

One of the most dangerous things about obsession is that it steals time we are supposed to be dedicating to other things. My husband would often look me in the eye and say, "You have to slow down, you have to be home more, you have to be here with me and not in la la land!" The truth was, I tended to go there a lot! See, if you are overdoing it at work, there is a chance you will become very irritable at home, possibly be late in prepping your meals and forget to lay out an outfit for the next day and for lack of a better term, show up to work in "rags." This is a metaphor for life, people! You've heard of people running themselves ragged? Well, it happens. We let it happen. And then we complain and become unbearable. Overindulgence leads us to try to overcompensate and, oftentimes, leads to being overwhelmed. What started out as a healthy goal can have the reverse effect and take us further from what we're striving to achieve!

We can even be over-the-top when it comes to God. I know someone who scares others away by bombarding them with religious references—every situation calls for a biblical quote and every sentence ends with "Praise the Lord!" I am not saying that is wrong, because the word of God is healthy for our spirit, but when we force it on others it can have the reverse effect. It ruins the relationship between the people, and between them and God. And God doesn't want that for us!

In my journey to becoming divinely fit, I came to believe that God wants us to respect ourselves enough to balance and moderate what we put in our body, what comes out of our mouth, even how we act and react in all circumstances in order to maintain the balance in our everyday life. If you knowingly choose not to seek balance, then you are consciously making a choice to endure the pressure of imbalance.

> If you knowingly choose not to seek balance, then you are consciously making a choice to endure the pressure of imbalance.

By simply empowering the spirit with the truth—namely, that overindulgence of any kind is unnecessary and has consequences—you can move forward responsibly, with conscious decision-making, self-control, and a healthy balanced life. I often tell the participants of my Operation Drop It Program that they should use the time to learn about their bodies—what works with and against it. Once they reach goal weight they will be able to indulge responsibly and manage their eating and drinking in a conscious—versus—careless way. They must hold themselves accountable in order to stay committed to maintaining balance in their everyday lives.

What will you do with the awareness and choice to seek and maintain spiritual, mental, and physical balance? This decision will help you get closer to becoming divinely fit.

SPIRIT-MIND-BODY EXERCISE

SPIRIT: When tempted to return to old patterns and behaviors, recite the mantra, "I am conscious of balance" or the prayer, "God, be my center and balance." Identify something that you are currently overindulging in that has had a direct consequence on your life, goals, et cetera.

MIND: Create at least 3 safety measures (i.e. find accountability partners; hide credit cards; do not buy certain items for your home; walk away when people start gossiping; set alarms to ensure time limits; leave a note on the scale to "only weigh on Wednesday," and so on) that help control the temptation to overindulge.

BODY: Do 15 jump squats every time you need to recite the above mantra or prayer.

The Struggle
with the Temple

Do you not know that your bodies are temples of the Holy
Spirit, who is in you, whom you have received from God? You
are not your own; you were bought at a price.
Therefore honor God with your bodies.
Corinthians 6:19-20

There were plenty of times in my life when I abused my body. I hardly thought of my body as a temple and at times I even remember hating it. As a tween and teen I toyed with both starvation and bulimia; in my adult years I tried numerous workout fads including diet pills and lotions (I even sprinkled that crazy powder over my food!)— anything that promised instant results. All the while, I was still eating junk food and drinking three cups of café a day—light and sweet. Due to a family history of addiction I stayed away from mood-enhancing drugs and never imagined that my extreme behaviors around weight were also a form of addiction! Deep down, I knew the way I felt about my body wasn't right; I knew I should be grateful for it. I knew there were plenty of people who would love and appreciate the body I was in. I was just not there with myself.

For a long time, I even questioned what kind of person I was to have these thoughts and feelings. Eventually, though, I realized how common it was (especially for women) to be dissatisfied with one's body. Of course, these expectations are always based on fluctuating social norms. Back in the day, everyone wanted to be super-slim, with tiny butts. Now my daughter asks me what kind of exercises she can do to make her butt *bigger*! And no matter how many times I tell her that most of those bodacious backsides are fake and that a one-hundred-pound young lady would have to make squatting and lunging her life to obtain it, she remains enamored with oversized lips, breasts, and backsides. She's not alone. These days, it seems everyone is getting some-thing injected, augment-ed, cut, nipped, and tucked on the outside, but my question is, what about the inside? Now, I want to be clear—some people need/want surgery and do it in alignment with their spirit-mind-body process, and kudos to them. Most tend to be humbled by their surgery and are supportive of those "in the grind" (losing one pound at a time). Then there are those who have surgery for the wrong reasons, without regard for the temple they reside in and to the detriment of their spirit. Until they accept and acknowledge that the body is a temple created by God, most will continue to take it for granted, fall slave to cultural dictates, and engage in behaviors that make them feel helpless and desperate to be just like someone else.

> *It is super important that you find your own "feel good recipe," as it is the only way to truly honor the temple that you will live in the rest of your life.*

It took me quite some time to learn this valuable lesson, though I learned it real quick once I entered the fitness world, which is even more brutal than the culture at large. If you do not look a certain way, how could anyone believe you take classes at a studio, let along teach at one? It is definitely an added pressure that most fitness instructors suffer in silence. I know, because I did for years, until I figured out my personal "feel good recipe." These days, I live by the Whole 30 regimen; I work out at least five days a week and have integrated more yoga and breathwork into each workout. I see my chiropractor at least twice a week and get a massage once a month. Since I am at goal weight I sometimes indulge on the weekends on something sweet or an alcoholic beverage, but I always have a payback plan scheduled. I weigh myself daily and drink as much water as I can (this is a personal struggle of mine). I bathe with organic body scrubs, lather up with organic lotion and spray my room or linens with lavender or lemongrass. I do my nails bi-weekly and do pedicures bi-weekly in the summer and monthly in the winter (you should never completely stop!). I get a haircut every two weeks and dye the grays every six to eight weeks. I take apple cider vinegar, magnesium, glucosamine, adrenal support, and vitamins C and B daily. Oh, and I poop regularly (and you should too)! Most importantly, I have integrated prayer and meditation into my daily routine; I recite mantras and read as much as I can. It is super important that you find your own "feel good recipe," as it is the only way to truly honor the temple that you will live in the rest of your life. The specifics are up to you, but it means eating healthy, moving your body, hard work, commitment, consistency, treating yourself right, and giving yourself permission to dance freely in the temple the Creator has gifted you with. It is the way He destined it to be.

SPIRIT-MIND-BODY EXERCISE

SPIRIT: Recite the mantra, "My body is a temple" or the prayer, "God, thank you for making my body a sacred temple. I will do my best to treat it well."

MIND: Find your "feel good recipe." Make a list of things that when done consistently make you feel and look amazing. Now rate your commitment to each on a scale of 1 to 10, ten indicating the highest level of commitment. Next, write down what you can do improve each score, then take out a calendar and select dates to have each done by. If you have time, schedule some appointments (i.e. nails, massage). If you are lost and don't know where to start, dig a little deeper, ask friends or email me!

BODY: Drop into a wide squat and jump into and out of Goddess pose. Make sure your shoulders are back and you are inhaling and exhaling with every jump as a reminder of the Goddess our Lord created you to be. Recite the mantra or prayer with each repetition.

The Struggle with Conformity

Do not be conformed to this world,
but be transformed by the renewal of your mind,
that by testing you may discern what is the will of God,
what is good and acceptable and perfect.
Romans 12:2 ESV

Breaking into the fitness world in Connecticut in the mid-1990s was a very difficult thing. Back then, most fitness instructors were either blonde, blue-eyed women, sized 0 to 2, or perfect chiseled white or African American men. Then there was me: a caramel-colored Puerto Rican who wore a size 6. I did have one very important thing going for me, though: I was fired up to teach.

I can remember showing up to my first kickboxing certification dressed all in black, with a bandana on my head and an off-the-shoulder shirt I had designed and cut myself. This was my style at the time. When I walked in, one of the women said to me, "Do you know where you are going? This is a fitness certification." I just smiled and informed her that I was there to participate. With a chuckle, she handed me the information packet, then, as I walked away, tossed a "good luck" over her shoulder. I got a similar reaction when I entered a room full of people who definitely looked the part. They stared, smirked, and whispered as I took a long walk across the room to put my things down. The entire walk, I questioned myself. Why was I even there? I began to feel uncomfortable in the clothes I was in and then even in my own skin. At that time, I wanted nothing more than to conform to this world I had stepped into. In my head, conforming would make all these feelings go away.

As part of the certification process, we were broken down into groups. "You will have to memorize two combinations," the instructor informed us, "and make up two of your own." This made me feel even more uncomfortable; now, not only would my appearance be on display, but my choreography as well. Just then, I heard one of the women in my group whisper to another, "Ha, what is she about to do?" This could have made me pick up my things and leave, but instead it set off a light bulb in my head. Why was I even trying to fit into this world? I was who I was. I dressed how dressed. I walked and moved how I walked and moved. This was a test for me. A test that would discern what was truly good, acceptable, and perfect for me and no one else. It was in that instant that I invited God to let His will be done. When my name was called, I turned to the young ladies and whispered, "I will tell you what I am about to do—I am going to smoke this test as God has destined me to do." Only a small number finished the certification that day and, thankfully, I was one of them.

We've all compared ourselves to others at some point or another, and at some point, we've all felt that we came up short. The important question to ask is, what is the standard by which we measure ourselves? Who determines what success is, what it could be and/or should be? Are we playing by society's rules when we should be playing by God's? What if your real test, purpose, and destiny is something completely different than what you thought? And, finally, will you be so busy chasing someone else's success that you will never achieve the success that was meant for you? When I went for that certification I was a new mother and a full-time detective; I was also going to school and working out every day, usually for about two hours. Yet instead of acknowledging all of this, I was negatively comparing myself to those who had more fitness experience than me, looked differently than me, and perhaps had different resources than me. On some level I also felt this gave me the right to try to play copy-cat, with no regard for the process they had undergone to look the way they looked or be where they were.

It is not always easy, but with consistent effort (praying, self-talk, & checking in with yourself), you will be guided by the spirit, not comparison. You will be transforming, rather than conforming.

We are all being tested in this way, consciously and subconsciously. Everywhere we look—online, in magazines, or on the street, we are bombarded by examples of what we think we should be and have. "How come she graduated in only two years? It took me three"; "She has an expensive designer wardrobe, I shop at Kohl's"; "She has perfect lips and I have to paint mine on." In a blended home, it's "Why do his kids do or have (fill in the blank) when my kids only have (fill in the blank)?" If we're talking about weight loss, it's, "How come he lost fifty pounds in two months and it took me a year?" The list goes on and on, and if you aren't careful, making negative comparisons will take over your life.

The next time you find yourself comparing your life to another's, ask yourself, did you sign up for his/her process or are you just idolizing their result? Are you on your own journey or are you trying to make it what you think it "should" be, based on external forces? The fact is, when we're not firmly grounded in our spirit we allow the world to corrupt our authenticity by redefining our thoughts and actions. It is not always easy, but with consistent effort (praying, self-talk, and checking in with yourself), you will be guided by the spirit, not comparison. You will be transforming, rather than conforming. This is an essential piece of your journey to becoming divinely fit.

SPIRIT-MIND-BODY EXERCISE

SPIRIT: Recite this mantra, "I am imperfectly perfected," or this prayer: "Lord, thank You for anchoring me in a perfect spirit."

MIND: Name 2 people with whom you constantly compare yourself. Define them (nemesis, mentor, friend, et cetera). Write out the ways in which you compare yourself to them; then honestly evaluate whether you want the things they have and what you are willing to do to achieve them. Finally, figure out whether these comparisons are impacting you negatively or positively.

BODY: Do 20 lateral jumps (one foot and then the other) from side to side. One side is God and the other side is the physical world. Keep moving side to side until you cannot go anymore and consciously land on the God side, where you are perfect.

The Struggle with Forgiveness

Get rid of all bitterness, rage and anger, brawling and slander,
along with every form of malice. Be kind and compassionate
to one another, forgiving each other,
just as in Christ God forgave you.
Ephesians 4:31-32:

When I was twelve, I was molested by my mother's live-in boyfriend (we'll call him "Chester", as in "Chester the Molester"). One night, while I slept, Chester came into the room wearing nothing but a towel. I was awakened to him fondling me under my underwear while he masturbated. Even as my young mind minimized the experience, I knew I could not let it continue or, God forbid, escalate. The next day, I made it clear to this man and my mother that if he ever did that again, I would stab him to death without hesitation, and I meant it. From that night forward, I slept with a knife under my pillow in case I needed to protect myself or my younger sister. After that, my home life became very uncomfortable, to say the least. My mother did not want to believe what had happened, causing me to withdraw from her and placing a great strain on our relationship. Since it was clear Chester wasn't going anywhere, I took every precaution. I kept my sister with me as much as possible and found places we could go so as not to be in the house with Chester. When I was home, no matter how hot it was outside, I was fully clothed from head to toe, usually in a sweat suit. I was often hit for not talking or responding to Chester, which was painful not only physically but emotionally as well. Over the next few years I learned many unfavorable things about this man—and his other victims—and yet he continued to be a part of our lives. My mother and Chester eventually married, then, just as I was entering high school, their relationship fell apart and Chester moved on to another family. He was gone, but my feelings of anger and betrayal remained. They hardened my heart and became part of my persona.

When Paula Abdul came out with the song, "Cold-hearted Snake," everyone used to say she was talking about me. I know now that my mind had taken over, standing guard over my spirit and body. It was the only way I was able to suppress all the feelings around the Chester incident and everything that followed.

For years, this coping mechanism worked. I grew up, became a police officer, and was living my life. Everything was all good. Then, one day while on patrol I stopped by my mom's house to grab something to eat. I remember like it was yesterday parking my cruiser in the driveway, walking up the stairs, opening the door and

> We will feel compelled to do our best to forgive as we are forgiven and understand that others will fall short of our expectations, just as we fall short every single day.

hearing an all-too-familiar male voice echoing from the kitchen. Chester! I didn't know what he was doing there after all this time, but instantly, every feeling—the ones I'd dealt with, the ones I hadn't, and even a few new ones—boiled to the surface. I froze in my tracks, unable to move, unable to believe my ears. I asked God for the strength to leave, to set aside the very real desire to hurt this man. God granted me that prayer, though I don't remember leaving, just gasping for air as I shed tears of anger and uncontrollable rage. How could he do this to me? How could *she*? Suddenly, God spoke to my spirit. It dawned on me that had it not been for this experience I would not have had a need to go into law enforcement. I also realized that if not for the emergence of my "cold-hearted snake" character, I would not have made it to where I was in life. It had allowed me to get through high school, college, and the police academy. More importantly, it had enabled me to archive my trauma, without the need for therapy, and actually use it as fuel to protect and serve others, as well as myself. What really blew my mind, though, was the realization that I needed to go through the experience of hearing Chester in my mother's kitchen in order to appreciate what God had done in my life. Furthermore, I believe it was a test of my ability to withdraw from bitterness, anger, and pain, and to initiate forgiveness.

For me, part of this process was to try to understand why they had acted and reacted as they did. In the course of my "research," I found out that Chester had been sexually, physically, and verbally abused himself. And my mother, well, I believe she was seeking love in all the wrong places and doing the best she could with what she knew at the time. God allowed me to see it this way and eventually forgive them. It wasn't easy, but whenever I doubted my ability to forgive I would think of God and how He forgives us of our sins each day. We are quick to judge and fire back at those that hurt us, but if we approach hurtful situations in the spirit, we will rest in the truth that no one is perfect. We will feel compelled to do our best to forgive as we are forgiven and understand that others will fall short of our expectations, just as we fall short every single day. If we are not compassionate with each other we risk complete solitude and invite pain and suffering to remain the primary focus of our everyday lives. Part of being divinely fit rests on our spirit being free, and freedom of the spirit requires us to release all "bitterness, rage and anger, brawling and slander, along with every form of malice." This test of faith requires us to ignore the flesh and instead act in the spirit. Seek freedom from the ego and enjoy the release of the pains and scars of the past. If nothing else has worked, this is definitely worth a try.

SPIRIT-MIND-BODY EXERCISE

SPIRIT: Whenever situations arise that cause (old or new) bitterness or hurt to surface, recite this mantra, "Let it go," or prayer, "Lord, help me forgive others as I am forgiven."

MIND: Make a list of people that you have not forgiven for incidents that occurred in the past or are currently happening. Then order them according to how long they have been present in your life. If you are still speaking to the person, ask yourself what takes more out of you: to forgive them or to hold onto your anger or hurt feelings. If you are not on speaking terms, ask yourself whether it hurts you more to reach out or to continue the estrangement. Once you answer this question, and assuming it is possible and preferable to reach out, you can then determine if sending a letter, email, text, or phone call is best. (If the person has passed away or you do not want to contact them you can write the letter then tear it up, burn it, et cetera.) This is not necessarily about reestablishing a relationship, but about letting the other person know that you forgive them, no strings attached. Remember, the purpose of this communication is not to get a response, but to free your own spirit with an act of forgiveness.

BODY: Do 10 burpees while reciting the above mantra or prayer. Repeat as needed.

The Struggle with Envy

A tranquil heart gives life to the flesh,
but envy makes the bones rot.
Proverbs 14:30

After going to a particular fitness convention for many years, I applied to be a presenter and was shocked when they turned me down. I was certain I deserved to be on that stage, and the fact that the "powers that be" disagreed had me twisted! I believe my ego was hurt and it called out some sort of envy. We have all struggled with envy at some point in our lives; this bears out in scientific research, which has found that envy is a natural human response to certain life events. The important thing is how we deal with those thoughts. Do we normally handle them in the spirit? Or, do we let our mind fester with negativity? Do we communicate envy with our body (facial expressions, mannerisms, sighs, et cetera.)? Envy can hang out in the mind for a hot second but then it's time for your spirit to takeover and go to work! Being honest with ourselves is hard, but it can prevent us from saying or doing things we will regret. Resting in God and His promise to provide us with a tranquil heart prevents us from letting these feelings rot in our spirit, mind, and body, creating dark roots in the core of our being.

Ironically, many years later the same convention held a "So You Think You Can Present" competition and I decided our team would enter. This time my intent was spirit-driven, about God's mission to touch lives through me and how I could use my gifts to inspire instructors to be the best they could be for the people they serve. I also made it very clear to my team that, win or lose, our presentation would fill the room with an authentic vibe...and that it did. We won first place and many praises from the judges. It felt so amazing because I knew God was at the forefront. The experience would also provide confirmation that my spirit had changed. One of the perks of winning first place was a slot to present at the next convention; however, when that event rolled around, we watched as the second-place winner went on to present in our place, no explanation given. In the flesh, I was like, *why is this happening? We won. They owe us. We deserve it.* But in my spirit, I knew God had a reason for them to present instead of us. I also realized I didn't need that stage to continue my life's work. God had blessed me with many other opportunities and above all, a tranquil heart. I prayed for the amazing presenters to come and fulfill their purpose, year after year, on that stage. When I recently heard that the convention had been dissolved I was genuinely saddened. I chose to focus, not on what we were not given, but more on the valuable lessons we learned and the amazing people we met in all the years we attended. The point is, we are constantly presented with opportunities to cultivate a tranquil heart or the rotting bones that continue to decay our spirit. The choice is yours.

Without a tranquil heart, envy and jealousy are guaranteed, as is the resulting stress, anxiety, depression, and anger it will cause your mind and body. When envious of others, you are relinquishing control of your spirit, mind, and body to others, and to material pursuits. Do you think the girl holding that Louis Vuitton bag knows you're going to go home, curl up in a ball and cry because you wanted the same bag for so long? No, she is enjoying the fruits of her labors, because she worked her butt off to get it. Do you believe that the couple dancing lovingly in front of you has no issues? Well, unbeknownst to you this is the first time they've been out since burying their child and are trying to forget their pain for a few hours! Do you wish you could buy the perfect body shape or dieting quick fix, without taking into ac-count the need for

> *Minimize envy's role in your life and maximize the God's manuscript, which carries with it everything you could ask for, and more.*

hard work and commitment? Do you see now how ridiculous it is to envy something when you really don't know the story behind it? Minimize envy's role in your life and maximize God's manuscript, which carries with it everything you need, and more.

As I mentioned earlier, envy is a normal human emotion. Left unchecked, it can make us crazy, irrational, and in its extreme, suicidal, or homicidal. But when we give it to God, He will help us get our minds right, away from the negative thoughts and closer to the truth of our many blessings. Envy not only affects people individually; it also divides and conquers, preventing us from working together and learning from, supporting, and loving each other. It is for this reason that I pray daily and specifically for humankind, that we all can set our envy aside. Remember, envy should play no part in the story of your life. Sure, it will show up for an audition, but it is your job to give your spirit the starring role.

SPIRIT-MIND-BODY EXERCISE

SPIRIT: Recite the word Namaste` as your mantra for the

day. This word means "the light in you reflects the light in me." When you honor this light in another, it gives you permission to shine with a tranquil and peaceful heart, with no room for envy. You can also pray, "God, Your peace is upon me."

MIND: Write down the names of at least 3 people you envy and the reasons why. If the reason for your envy is material, ask yourself whether you truly need or want the object (is it really as desirable as it appears to be?). If so, ask yourself, is it attainable? If it's not currently attainable, does the desire for it push you to a new level? Now, rate, on a scale of 1 to 10, how serious the envy is. How does it make you feel and how long does it take you to get over it? Most importantly, does it rob you of your authenticity, as opposed to a tranquil heart, which allows your authenticity to emerge?

BODY: Sit on the floor with your back against the wall. Draw your knees in toward your chest, a couple of inches away. Rest your arms down by your side with your chin slightly elevated toward the ceiling. Recite the mantra or prayer, then breathe in for 4 seconds and exhale for 4 seconds. Repeat at least 4 times.

The Struggle with Bitterness

For I see that you are in the gall of bitterness and
in the bond of iniquity.
Acts 8:23 ESV

Like most of us, I have seen and experienced the gall of both bitterness and iniquity. They share similarities yet there are distinct differences in the way they control us individually, collectively, and culturally. I know a man who refused to look within himself when his marriage fell apart, then watched his bitterness consume him and seep into his relationship with his children. Sadly, no matter how much his ex-wife tried to bolster them, they always seemed to return to the bitterness passed onto them. The point to this story? Bitterness can be passed from generation to generation unless someone holds themselves accountable and chooses to break the cycle.

Back in the day, I was known for cutting off people who hurt me without a second thought. I even had a term for it, "trimming the fat." My thought was, why should I submit myself to carrying extra fat around when I had the power to lose it? What I didn't realize was that my "trimming the fat" process was rooted in bitterness, a sort of "gangsta" mentality, like the offending person or thing would be dead to me. It seemed prudent, even amusing, at the time, but when I think of it now it seems pretty awful. I realize it was a dog-eat-dog (external) mentality, rather than a spiritual (internal) one. I justified my thoughts and actions by telling myself that I had to do what was needed as a matter of survival. This life lesson remains a struggle for me; there are still times when my head wants to spin off my body like "The Exorcist" and I have to pray myself out of a nasty thought or reaction. For me, active prayer and calling on my spirit saved me and many others.

I have found that bitterness is evil, bold, and relentless, and it can control a person's mind at any given time. It can take root for a second, a minute, an hour, a day, a month, a season, a year, a decade, or your entire life—the choice is yours. Are you mad because you didn't finish high school or college? Or that someone else always gets the "big breaks"? Or that so-and-so has it all and you don't? What stories are you telling yourself about the unfairness of life? I ask this because almost everything we perceive about ourselves, our lives, and the world is a story we've created in our minds; we then edit and re-edit these stories and give them multiple endings. They're like some trashy tabloid magazine, containing little to no truth but still manage to rile you up something fierce. See, bitterness sparks and awakens our ego and pride. It's called an overloaded ego boost. Then, it blurs the lines of your personal destiny. If bitterness takes root, it takes the opportunity to grow into a bittersweet nothing.

> *Above all, bitterness perpetuates unfair and immoral behavior because it is not rooted in LOVE.*

Bitterness takes hostages and places them in mental— and sometimes physical—bondage. This bondage is also both internal (meaning we're wicked (unfair) to ourselves) and external (meaning we're wicked to others. Internal bondage is silent on the outside and loud on the inside. It is fierce, and it is real, because we recreate it every day. Being wicked to others, however, is a type of bondage that is loud and applauded on the outside and silent on the inside. Both types of bondage stem from inner conflict and leave us with seemingly insurmountable guilt, which in turn leads to more bondage. It can cause rifts among family members and friends, destroy marriages, and even create a "mob mentality" of hate toward people and/or groups we don't even know. Above all, bitterness perpetuates unfair and immoral behavior because it is not rooted in LOVE. The spirit has no room for bitterness, however, it can live in the mind and body for as long as you allow it to.

Before you can deal with bitterness, you have to respect its sheer audacity, and understand its bond to unfairness, immorality, and wickedness. It is also quite sneaky and insidious and will creep back into your mind and heart if you're not vigilant. Though I've had a lot of victories in this area, there are still times when I throw my hands up and say, "God, you handle this because I can feel my bitterness creeping up like heartburn." Yes, it is that serious and my awareness minimizes it, but does not eliminate, the threat. I am still a work in progress and under construction year-round. Many of us walk around as if we don't know that bitterness has a hold on some part of our lives, but we do. When the bitter fire inside you begins to burn, the only way to put it out is to call out to the spirit of God—our living water. When you do, know that all your guilt and iniquities have been washed away. Yes, each day will still be a challenge, and it will take practice, but I am a firm believer that with commitment and consistency to be spirit-driven, the fires of bitterness within the mind and body will be extinguished.

SPIRIT-MIND-BODY EXERCISE

SPIRIT: Recite the mantra, "Bitterness will not control me" or the prayer, "God, continue to release me from my personal bondage."

MIND: Examine your heart and mind for things, people, and/or situations that have caused or are causing bitterness to take root in your life. List 5 (you could write them on a sticky note and even take a photo and make it your screensaver) and put it somewhere you'll be sure to see it. Each day, reflect on the list and ask yourself whether your bitterness holds you back from happiness in certain areas of your life. Make a conscious effort to start your day by welcoming God's spirit into those areas in an effort to release you from bondage.

BODY: Run in place for 2 minutes (using a timer and doing your best not to stop) while reciting the above mantra or prayer. This run represents leaving bitterness behind.

The Struggle with Judgment

Do not judge by appearances,
but judge with right judgment.
John 7:24 ESV

Most of us have struggled with judgment at one point or another. We are taught not to judge others, yet every day we are bombarded with standards (some fair, some unrealistic) against which we are to measure appearance, behavior, social status—the list goes on and on. There have been many instances in my own life when judgment was an issue—I have been both the judger and the one being judged. As a rookie cop, I was judged by the community in which I served, not only because of my five-foot-three-inch stature, but because I was a familiar face (I had grown up there). I also remember my supervisors and, in some instances, my fellow officers, judging whether or not I was qualified to be on the job, based solely on the fact that I was female. On the flip side, I have also judged people based on all sorts of things. While on the job, I had to size people up (in essence, judge them) because my life depended on making quick decisions based on what I knew at the time of an encounter. And frankly, 99.9% of the time I was dead-on. Such is the nature of being a cop. There were, however, a handful of times when I was *dead wrong*. One example is when I was a detective in the Intelligence Unit. We were doing surveillance in a very hot drug spot (a predominantly Spanish and Afro-American neighborhood with a predominately Caucasian clientele) and had been making back-to-back narcotics arrests. So, when we saw a car driven by a thin, frazzled, disheveled, nervous white male—along with other telltale factors—we definitely had "reasonable suspicion" (the legal standard) to pull him over. This was confirmed—or so we thought—when we found several vials of what appeared to be liquid PCP in his possession. Imagine our shock when we discovered that he turned out to be a Mormon priest, delivering holy water as a blessing to the drug dealers in the community! While this may seem humorous now, it certainly wasn't in the moment. As for the priest, he understood that we'd made a judgment call based on our training, experience, and the facts as they appeared to us. Before he drove away, he said, "Your hearts were in the right place and you were right to judge. I knew I hadn't done anything wrong." These powerful words resonated with me long after he had gone, and they resonate with me to this day. They remind me to examine my heart when judging others to ensure that it is not done with ill will.

Ironically, it seemed that the closer I came to that truth, the more I was judged by others. This was especially true when I added "fitness instructor" to my resume. Suddenly, everything from what I wore to class or in a photo to how I cut my hair was a topic of discussion. What folks loved to talk about most was my weight (specifically whether I was up ten pounds or down ten pounds) and what I ate in public. I can distinctly remember going to a Jack-n-Jill celebration and my husband alerting me to an entire table watching my every move. At that time, I was eating a salad (I do love a good salad) which I chose over other food items because I had made a conscious decision to save my calories for a couple cocktails—anyone who knows me knows I would rather have a cocktail than mashed potatoes and would pass on pasta to have a piece of my *prima's* cake. As I ate, I heard their whispers, I could feel their shaming eyes burning into the back of my head. Then, in an impulsive (and not very ladylike) moment I plucked a cupcake from the stand, turned around to face the table, raised the cupcake up to my mouth and licked it several times, all while engaging them in full eye contact. You could almost hear their gasp over the music as they tried to look away but just couldn't. In the flesh, their judgment bothered me

> It is only by anchoring ourselves in the spirit and holding our minds and mouths accountable that we will be able to determine the true nature of our judgmental thoughts.

tremendously; these days, when I view such things in the spirit, I see them as irrelevant. I also understand that their judgment comes from their own wounds and scars and are subconsciously rooted in envy and jealousy, a reflection of their own perceived shortcomings.

Knowing that I was being judged so harshly helped me lean on my spirit when I was being judged and learn not to judge others in the same way. The key is taking the time to be right with your judgment. Are you judging a person or situation based on ill will or jealousy, or are you using healthy discernment based on facts, experience, and divine guidance? It is only by anchoring ourselves in the spirit and holding our minds and mouths accountable that we will be able to determine the true nature of our judgmental thoughts. The truth is, if we were not there to witness someone's process, how can we judge what we perceive as the result? And even if we do witness the process, who are we to judge? Imagine if God chose to judge us for all that we did, knowingly and unknowingly! Refresh your spirit, mind, and body in the truth: we should offer people what God offers us, a judgment-free zone.

As you grow closer to becoming divinely fit, you'll notice judgmental thoughts, both toward yourself and others, becoming less prominent in your life. It is imperative that you get a grip on your negative thoughts; if you let them consume you, they will keep you on the sidelines while life passes you by.

SPIRIT-MIND-BODY EXERCISE

SPIRIT: Recite this mantra, "This is a judgment-free zone" or the prayer "God, free me from judgment of myself and others."

MIND: Think back over your day. How many times did you say or think judgmental things toward yourself and/or others? Assess the situation(s). Do you believe you were right to judge? If you're having a hard time figuring it out, ask yourself whether you like to be judged in this manner. The goal here is not to judge yourself for being judgmental; it is to ground yourself in the truth that all humans are imperfect.

BODY: When you need to release judgment toward yourself and/or others, do 20 right-to-left lunges while reciting the above mantra or prayer.

The Struggle Between Mind and Spirit

But Daniel resolved not to defile himself with the royal food and wine, and he asked the chief official for permission not to defile himself this way… 'Please test your servants for ten days: Give us nothing but vegetables to eat and water to drink. Then compare our appearance with that of the young men who eat the royal food and treat your servants in accordance with what you see.' At the end of the ten days they looked healthier and better nourished than any of the young men who ate the royal food.
Daniel 1:8, 12, 13, 15

As clearly stated in the above scripture, the Bible draws a comparison between a healthy lifestyle and our outward appearance. Moreover, nutritional experts and medical experts since the beginning of time have acknowledged that consuming vegetables and plenty of water is the best way to look and feel your best. Yet, incredibly, even today, many people have a hard time believing that there is a direct connection between what they put in their bodies and what they see in the mirror. If you're one of those people, all the facts are just a quick Google search away. But research is only the first step; you also have to believe it, and most importantly, you have to *apply* it. Right now you may be thinking *easier said than done* and I am saying, I agree with you. I know for a fact it's not easy, because I have lived it. As humans, we naturally want what is appealing to the eyes *and* delicious to the tongue, even if it defies the truth that is grounded in our spirit.

This truth is that we do not NEED unhealthy food, we WANT it. Our appearance is therefore the outgrowth of our choices, both conscious and unconscious. Now, I acknowledge that these choices are affected by the culture we're born into and the environment we grow up in. My exposure to various cultures and cuisines created a love for food in general, some of them unhealthy. I didn't think much about it until about 2010, when a nutritionist buddy challenged me to give up my coffee, or, as I affection-

> *When you fall off the wagon, the key is not to judge or beat yourself up about it, but to regroup and recommit yourself to making choices that are conscious and completely transparent among the spirit-mind-body.*

ately call it, *mi café*. Actually, she didn't really challenge me; she just brought it to my attention that if I did abstain I could lose those extra five to ten pounds I had been struggling with—just like many others do. Back then I drank mi café light and sweet (like me) and I admit that each Fall I looked forward to adding the pumps of yummy pumpkin flavor. Not surprisingly, I didn't want to hear my friend's advice. See, mi café had been a part of my life since I could remember. When I did give it up for a year and a half, I indeed lost those excess pounds, not just because of the café but because the choice I'd made prompted me to make other healthy choices as well. I came to the conclusion that I didn't need mi café, I simply wanted it. It was a habit. When I did resume drinking it, I had a different mindset: I used regular cream and no sugar unless it was coconut sugar. With this simple change I was able to enjoy mi café in my regimen without it affecting my weight.

Years later, I, along with the nutritionist at my studio, researched, tried, endured, and adopted the Whole 30 regimen as part of our famously successful Operation Drop It program and support group. One of the program parameters is no sugar or dairy, so as difficult as it was, I tried mi café with almond creamer and no sugar and drank it like that for quite some time. The point is, this program helped me further distinguish my food needs from my wants, and further define what worked for my body. Most importantly, it helped me put into perspective what foods were worth the internal and external consequences.

To this day, most of my food and drink choices are made in strict adherence to the Whole 30 regimen...with the exception of mi café. My weekends do vary but are paired with payback workouts for the foods that are not Whole 30-compliant. At this stage in my life, my spirit's truth allows me to consciously make choices that my mind and body can live with, and it feels awesome. That said, I am now at my goal weight, and therefore have greater freedom from which to negotiate my food and beverage choices. Sometimes I choose the alcoholic beverage or the pumpkin cake, but not both unless I have a plan in place. If I slip out of my five-pound range after a series of bad choices (conscious or not), I gather myself together and go back to hard work. Right now you may be wondering, "Does this still happen to her?" Well, the answer is, "Yes, it happens to everyone except Jesus." When you fall off the wagon, the key is not to judge or beat yourself up about it, but to regroup and recommit yourself as quickly as you can to making choices that are conscious and completely transparent among the spirit-mind-body. These are the choices that leave you with no regrets. I am not talking about fad diets, but about sustainable daily choices that form the basis of a healthy lifestyle. If you do the legwork and discover what really works for your body, it will be much easier to permanently incorporate them into your life. Feed your mind with the spirit and your body with those veggies and I promise you will see results! Let God be your nourishment guide and you will find your road to becoming divinely fit much smoother.

SPIRIT-MIND-BODY EXERCISE

SPIRIT: Rely on the spirit to help you discern what you need versus what you want. Re-read Daniel's commitment to not defile his spirit-mind-body and use the mantra, "I am consciously choosing to serve my need/want." Note how admitting it makes you feel. Or, pray, "Lord, help me serve my needs and not my wants."

MIND: Google the Whole 30 grocery list, then list 5 foods you eat each day that are not on that list. Out of those 5, pick 2 and omit them from your diet for a week to see how your mind and body feel. Or, do you best to commit to drinking 4 bottles of water each day. Journal one or both efforts and see what positive changes come from it.

BODY: Do 20 power jacks to get your mind right and your heart pumping as you recite the above mantra and/or prayer.

The Struggle with Humility

For everyone who exalts himself will be humbled,
and he who humbles himself will be exalted.
Luke 14:11 ESV

It is not always easy to remain humble. We all want recognition for our achievements, we want to be seen. Sometimes, though, our need to be exalted takes over our lives, rules our hearts, and hurts us and others. If you're facing this battle, know that you are not alone. It is one that has existed since the beginning of time. It is part of the human condition. Indeed, Christ's humility is one of the qualities people most want to emulate and have the hardest time with. We must talk about humility if we want to personally emulate it and collectively grow it.

I have seen people exalt themselves in ways that degrade, depress, ridicule, and make fools of others. I have seen mothers and fathers neglect their children or treat them horribly, then exalt themselves through the kids' accomplishments. I have seen supervisors work their people like dogs, steal their ideas, and exalt themselves. I have seen people in the fitness industry lose their authenticity and step on their colleagues and clients to rise to the top. I have seen people take shortcuts to weight loss and exalt themselves over those who embrace the grind and work at it day by day. I have seen people pay others to do their schoolwork and exalt themselves when they graduate. I have seen non-profit agencies steal money, misrepresent statistics, and exalt themselves for achieving "results." I have seen friends and family bask in the misfortune of their loved ones to make themselves feel better, and if I have seen it, then I am sure you've seen it too.

On the other hand, I have also seen incredible humility, often from some of the most successful, and unsuccessful, people around. When I hear about the attitude and actions of such people, be they famous athletes or actors, entrepreneurs, or homeless people, I take the time to learn more about their story and I usually discover that they are deeply spiritual people. It seems that those who live in the spirit don't need to take credit for others' work. Instead, they seek to exalt others, and their connection with them is effortless.

If you and I have seen all of this, rest assured that God has seen it as well. What does that mean? It means that those who humble themselves will be exalted and those who exalt themselves will be humbled at some point in their lives. This is what is referred to as "karma" or "eating humble pie." I don't know about you, but I'd rather make a conscious choice to be humble than be humbled by circumstance.

Growing up, I was perceived to be the favorite because I excelled in school, participated in sports, and was a rule follower. This gave my mom easy bragging rights because I was often being recognized for some sort of achievement, but at the same time it alienated me from my siblings resulting in feelings of loneliness and my subsequent decision to minimize all my accomplishments. According to them, I was the favorite, but I felt I received no benefit for it. For example, I decided not to walk on stage to receive my bachelor's degree because I was the first one in my family to graduate college and I didn't want to draw attention (positive or negative) to myself. I truly believed that if I minimized myself and my accomplishments, I would make everyone around me feel better. In essence, I had learned by default *not* to exalt myself. I do not remember it being a choice—and I certainly didn't enjoy it—that was just was the way it was. However, this "built-in" humility became an asset during my spiritual awakening. Once I realized that Christ had entrusted all of us, including me, to be a vessel in His kingdom, I embraced being the center of attention, but it was all for His glory, not mine. It gave me the opportunity to showcase Christ as the amazing one and share how much He had changed my life. My goal became to present my business and life as an example to others, on a real and raw level they can relate to and be encouraged by.

> *A humble spirit can be the pathway to what you say and do. It will also allow you to lead by example and glorify God in the process.*

A humble spirit can be the pathway to what you say and do. It will also allow you to lead by example and glorify God in the process.

When your spirit is humble it guides your mind and body in a way that is beneficial to you and those around you. By minimizing your importance, you maximize the importance of others; it is reciprocated, and everyone wins. This begins at home, with the people we love; for example, my husband puts me first, I put him first, and we both benefit equally.

If you do your best to keep your spirit humble, you can rest assured that whatever comes your way comes for a reason. Have no fear, you will be exalted, not in your time, but in God's time. Stay focused on that truth and move forward, leaving no room in your life for arrogance. The fact is, your humble spirit reflects God's love and provides others with an example of what goodness should look like. This humility is a cornerstone to becoming divinely fit, which requires you to consistently ground yourself in the spirit, in an effort to empower the mind and body.

SPIRIT-MIND-BODY EXERCISE

SPIRIT: Recite the mantra "I chose to humble myself" or pray "God, today I will reflect Your humble heart."

MIND: List specific instances where you have been served a piece of humble pie. On a scale of 1-10 (1 being the least) rate your level of humility before these instances and after; this will help you gain perspective on your humbleness (or lack thereof) affects your life.

BODY: Do 20 squat jumps as you recite the above mantra or prayer and you will burn off the humble pie and keep it off.

The Promises

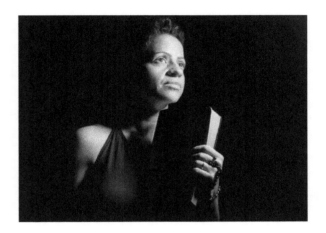

As children of the most-high God,
we have been promised the gifts of forgiveness,
acceptance, and unconditional love.
The following chapters define these promises and remind
us of our many opportunities to remain grounded in
divine light, as well as our responsibility to share that
light with others.

The Promise of God's Insurance Policy

No temptation has overtaken you except what is common to mankind. And God is faithful; He will not let you be tempted beyond what you can bear. But when you are tempted, He will also provide a way out so that you can endure it.
1 Corinthians 10:13

You don't need me to tell you that this world is brimming with temptation. It is everywhere we look— material objects, beautiful people, or the promise of glory. These temptations often spark conversations in our heads—these are the stories and lies we tell ourselves; they provide justification for giving into these temptations, even to the detriment of ourselves and others. When I worked in the police department, many men and women gave me all sorts of justifications for why they had been unfaithful. The consensus was that the temptation to be unfaithful became stronger when they met someone who seemed to have all the qualities their significant other did not. The more they spent time with that someone, the louder the thoughts, reasons, and justifications became until he/she seemed essential to happiness. I know, because this happened to me. The difference is that when I met that someone, I was able to forego the temptation and instead offered him an ultimatum and opportunity for a healthy blended family. I knew that if his feelings for me were as serious as mine were for him, he would back them up with action. If he didn't, he was not the man God intended me to be with. As it turned out, he was that man. He got a divorce, pursued me in earnest, and today we are happily married. To be clear, I am not justifying this situation; I am simply giving an example of what we can reap when we resist the temptation of the flesh and instead rely on the one who created us with value.

I also faced temptation at the workplace. When I became a police officer, I expected a fair amount of resentment from the male officers. What I did not expect was harsh treatment from other females. Some of them barely spoke to me, others picked on me for any little mistake I made, while others ridiculed me for being so young. Some of these women even resorted to telling lies about me and about other females in my academy class. At first, I was confused and hurt as to why this was happening, but then I realized that women were being pitted against each other. All females on the job were judged by any mistake, shortcoming, or character flaw displayed by one. And while it was true that some of the female cops slept around or were consistently out of work because they were injured or pregnant, many more consistently proved themselves to be serious-minded, capable, dedicated officers. After several years on the job and attaining a healthy level of respect among my fellow officers, I found myself tempted to treat the new females just as harshly as I had been treated. I told myself that I would be justified in doing so, that I would be "molding" these new officers just as I had been molded. I struggled with this temptation every time someone

> When the spirit leads and the mind gets on board with the body (in this case, your mouth) you can overcome any temptation.

gossiped about another female cop, especially if I knew the information to be true. I will even admit that at times I participated in the banter. Then it occurred to me that just because it had been done to me didn't give me the right to do it to someone else. From that moment on, I found the strength to resist the temptation; when someone started to trash a female officer, I bit my tongue, whether or not I liked her, and whether or not I knew the rumor was accurate.

Eventually, I took it a step further and called out the cavalry. "Do you know that to be true," I'd ask, "and if so, who are you to judge?" Needless to say, many of those conversations stopped taking place in front of me. I had turned my negative temptation into a positive action. On the other hand, the grapevine was helpful. I'd heard I was a little intimidating, so when new female officers came on the job, I made it a point to introduce myself and make myself available for counsel. I let them know I could be their mentor, not their tormentor!

Temptation is a normal part of life, and it's even stronger when we feel we have been wronged. However, when we rely on God, we realize that He always shows us another way. In the flesh, I might have wanted to join in the "hazing" of those women, but in the spirit, I knew I would best serve Him—and my fellow officers—by overcoming temptation and instead focusing on a positive course of action.

Temptation even shows up on your plate. Ask anyone who has struggled with weight and they will tell you there is no greater temptation than food. It is not just about taste, either; we are most tempted to overindulge when our emotions are riding high. I can remember battling with a row of Oreos after a bad day or attacking my "emergency chocolate bar" in one sitting, instead of eating it in small pieces as is intended. Food is also an equal opportunity temptation, difficult to resist when people are around (i.e. holidays) and when they're not (i.e. closet eating while spending time alone with our painful thoughts).

What we need to realize is that temptation and self-sabotage often go hand in hand. For no matter what the temptation is, the battle is not between ourselves and the object of our desire, but between us and our mind. I've spoken to many people who tell me how a particular food or beverage has so much power over them. How can this be? We know it is not good for us, yet we find ourselves locked in a struggle to resist. We try to justify eating it, telling ourselves that it's just one meal or snack, so what's the big deal? Or that we've had a bad day, week, et cetera, and deserve comfort, usually in the form of a drink or sugary treat. When we feel sorry for ourselves we are able to justify actions that we know down deep are not in our best interest. However, when we develop a transparent relationship among our spirit, mind, and body, the temptation lessens and sometimes even evaporates. Our needs are filled by the spirit and we no longer need to self-sabotage. What does this mean in the flesh? It means not putting the triple chocolate cake on the counter, so you can see it and be tempted every second you are in the kitchen. We are visual people, so minimize the visuals and concentrate on the spirituals!

You also need to realize that temptations—at least those in the form of food cravings—usually last no more than five minutes. In the flesh this can seem like five hours, but when you call on your spirit, you will see the truth: you will not be tempted beyond what you can handle. The spirit also knows it can endure the temptation. We simply must learn to focus not on our failures, but on our triumphs. When the spirit leads, and the mind gets on board with the body (in this case, your mouth) you can overcome any temptation. When we choose to acquire God's "insurance policy," we understand that we will never be tempted beyond our personal abilities. Temptations are simply part of the process of becoming divinely fit and, seen from a spiritual perspective serve as milestones on the journey to a healthier you.

SPIRIT-MIND-BODY EXERCISE

SPIRIT: Write this mantra, "Today, I will not be tempted beyond what I can bear" or prayer, "God, with Your strength I know I can endure or escape any temptation" on a sticky note and place it on your mirror, computer, or door (you can even make it your screensaver). This will help you walk in the spirit and deter your mind and body from indulging in negative temptations that present themselves to you throughout the day.

MIND: What are your largest temptations in life? How do you feel after you succumb to them? Write them down, along with what you perceive as your weaknesses. Circle two, and for one week, use the spirit exercise to gain strength in those areas.

BODY: Do 10 pushups as you recite the above mantra or prayer. The downward motion symbolizes the weight of the temptation bearing down on you. The upward motion symbolizes the strength you acquire from beating the temptation.

The Promise of Love

Whoever says he is in the light and hates his brother
is still in darkness.
1 John 2:9 ESV

There is no doubt that we are living in complicated and trying times. We are divided along racial and political lines and are increasingly pressured to "choose sides." Both sides think they are right and oftentimes confuse the will of man with the will of God. I have witnessed people preaching that they are God's people and that we should all "be love," all while spewing negativity and hate. Problems usually arise when a particular person, group, or side does not achieve their desired outcome. This is when the lines between entitlement, privilege, rights, and equality become blurred, and sometimes create a mob mentality that erupts in vulgar language and tumultuous violence. News flash: when this happens, it is not God's will, it is man's. So how can we more effectively voice frustration and combat inequality? The answer is *peacefully*. Let God and the love He shines on the world be your moral compass. And, yes, we are human and yes, we get angry. We must remember that He is in control. We must be slow to anger and present our case with grace, love, and humility.

I learned this lesson the hard way. For years, I fought battles, both within the police department and the Hartford community, by yelling and puffing my chest out. I called people names, sought revenge, and sometimes intentionally hurt others' feelings. Deep down I knew I was wrong because my spirit told me so, yet my mind still wanted to fight, fight, fight and show, show, show them that I could demolish them in one breath and without batting an eyelash. Yes, I had a reputation for "getting it done," but at the end of the day I didn't reflect God's love or His will. I reflected my own agenda, ego, pride, and—deep down—my own personal hurt and need to be understood.

When we don't have God in our lives, our moral compass is askew. I have watched some of my own family members cut each other up and out of each other's lives while treating strangers like royalty. We are not unique; in fact, it goes on in every family. Though most hunger for inclusion, they operate from a place of personal darkness, which is something we as their family cannot fix. Sometimes they even treat others badly as a coping mechanism or just a learned behavior, although it really doesn't matter why. The bottom line is, we cannot be of the light while holding our brother in darkness.

The good news is, no matter how bitter or hardened we may become, it can take just one person to crack our hearts open. For me, that person was my daughter. Before she came along I was a tough cookie and I vowed nothing would ever change that. Well, she did, and now I am a tough cookie with a mushy center. Having to care for my daughter (who was very sick as a toddler) and putting her needs at the top of my list, helped me create a clear pathway from selfishness to selflessness. Such is being a parent. However, we don't have to have children to find our way to the light—we need only embrace the wellspring of love within us. Science cannot explain the boundaries of this love, because it is limitless. No matter how arrogant we are, no matter how cold or crude our culture is, we only need love to survive and prosper. Even our resentful and divisive world cannot subdue the power of love. Why? Because, as stated in 1 Corinthians 13:4-8, "Love is patient and kind; love does not envy or boast; it is not arrogant or rude. It does not insist on its own way; it is not irritable or resentful; it does not rejoice at wrongdoing but rejoices with the truth. Love bears all things, believes all things, hopes all things, endures all things. Love never ends…" We are destined to be that gleaming lighthouse in the middle of the dark ocean.

Our job as a lighthouse in the world is to shine love and light on darkness wherever we find it. For example, there have been times when envy and hate shake their ugly heads in my weight loss group—even among the most successful members. I have been doing this for quite some time and have the gift of discernment, even with the most complex people. While some appear to be happy, walking around in their new healthy bodies, they are still operating from a place of envy and self-loathing. When someone acts superior to those who are struggling, I call that person out. I remind him/her that they were once fifty pounds heavier and at the drop of a hat they could be right back there. In truth, I am simply calling upon their spirit and

We are all freedom fighters and truth warriors in some way and for different causes, but learning that God's agenda is more important than ours will undoubtedly make the world a better place.

helping them align it with their mind and body. This alignment process is not just about weight loss, but every area of life. You can praise Jesus all day long but if your feet are not firmly planted in the spirit, hate and envy will grow in you. Left unchecked, your light will get dimmer and you will conform to the darkness you have harvested within you or those around you.

When we hold ourselves above others, we hold *everyone* back. Understand this: while each of us struggles in (at least) one area of life—you may struggle with a relationship and I may struggle with physical fitness—we all have only one goal: to walk in the light and share it with others. And if we keep our eyes on this prize, we will find ourselves living in the spirit and not from ego, pride, or divisiveness. Regardless of our reasons or how "right" we think we are, sharing a degrading post about ANYONE, standing with a group that chants hateful things, calling people names, and rallying up others to generate a hateful mob mentality does *not* reflect God's love. If you have taken part in such activities in the past, know that you are not alone. Take the time to evaluate your reasons and your actions in an effort to create a more loving action plan, then forgive yourself and move on. As you become more divinely fit, it will become easier to remove yourself from hateful conversations and associations. I am not saying you should bury your head in the sand or ignore situations you consider unjust; I am suggesting that you be mindful about what you say and how you say it. I stand before you a work in progress and ask that you join me in that group. In this group we hold each other accountable to what comes out of our mouths and what actions we take. For me, some days are amazing and some days I lose a battle or two. Walking in the light doesn't mean you'll never react badly to another or get sucked into nasty political debates; it just means you are more aware. The difference for me is that my heart is now grounded in the spirit. When a trying situation arises, I take a deep breath and pray for God to touch my heart and give me clarity, so that when I address others I do so in a way that reflects His mission and not my own. We are all freedom fighters and truth warriors in some way and for different causes but learning that God's agenda is more important than ours will undoubtedly make the world a better place. It takes a lot of active prayer and support, but we are all capable.

Our opinions can be firm or fluid; our beliefs can be compromised or affirmed; our voices can create a movement or destroy it. It all comes down to how we as individuals choose to use our voice and allow the process to unfold. In the flesh we have the ability to doom ourselves to darkness, but when we do our very best to address issues in the spirit there is no end to our power. This is the power of love, gifted to us by God, and it affirms His promise that in the end, the light will always blind the darkness.

SPIRIT-MIND-BODY EXERCISE

SPIRIT: When faced with a test in this area, recite the mantra, "I now choose to be the light instead of darkness" or pray, "God, empower me to be light despite how I feel right now."

MIND: Make an honest list of people, groups, places, or things that you hate, as well as the reasons for your hatred. Next, make note of how you express your feelings—is it with harsh words or shared social media posts? Ask yourself whether these feelings and activities add to or detract from your life. For example, if your goal is love and inclusion, are you being hypocritical? How can your words and deeds be adjusted to reflect God's love while working toward your goal (i.e. rebuilding relationships or joining a movement?) Keep a journal to hold yourself accountable.

BODY: Recite the above mantra or prayer as you do 50

quick forward front kicks (right to left); this will help you kick away frustration, get your adrenaline going and breathe your way back into light and calmness. Make sure to take super deep breaths. End by wrapping your arms around yourself in an assurance that love exists. Repeat as needed.

The Promise for the Lighthouse Keeper

He came as a witness, to bear witness about the light,
that all might believe through him. He was not the light,
but came to bear witness about the light.
John 1: 7-8:

When someone told me many years ago that I should write a book about my life, I nearly laughed out loud. To me, only actors, CEOs, political and spiritual leaders, and famous philanthropists—in other words, "important people"—wrote books. What could I possibly have to say? My life was boring. I forgot all about the suggestion, until years later when a second person said, "You know, you really have a lot to say. You should write a book." And again, I thought, I am not qualified to write a book and who would want to read it, anyway? This, despite the fact that my story had already been captured in a book called "Women Warriors" and I had blogged and written articles. I had even been featured in a children's book called "Little Miss Pickle," about an officer who challenges an alligator that bullies others in an enchanted garden. Somehow, my mind had bypassed these positive experiences and landed smack dab on the negative. You see, everything else in my life had been validated by a test, certification, diploma, et cetera. There was no piece of paper, however, that would prove I was qualified to share my story. That was a conclusion I would have to come to on my own, and until

I did, I wouldn't see it come to fruition.

In June of 2016, while at a fitness conference in Los Angeles I attended a lecture called "The Next Step"— meaning the next step in your career. I remember sitting there and asking God how I could more effectively touch lives in a way that would fulfill His purpose. I also remember thinking, this is bigger than the studio because the studio has limits and I knew I could not put a limit on God's purpose and plan for me. After two hours the lecture ended and I walked out, my hand sore from notetaking and my mind overwhelmed by all I had learned. I found a secluded area, sat on the floor, and began eating a snack, still deep in thought. When I was finished I had a half-hour before the next session and began weeding through my emails, deleting the junk, and flagging important messages. Suddenly, one leapt out at me. It was a publishing company called "Powerful You" and it said something like, "I have seen your work and believe you would be a good fit as one of our authors." After almost throwing up, I called my lifelines with excitement and shock. Then, just as quickly, the excitement

> *If we rewire our belief from "we work for the man" to "we work for God" then we will be witnesses for Him by walking, acting, and reacting with light to the natural disappointments we face within ourselves and in life.*

was replaced by the negative thoughts associated with not being "good enough." For the next few days I continued to mull over "the book thing," as I called it, only to archive it along with the many other things, projects, dreams, and wishes I could possibly complete "one day."

In July of 2017, while at another fitness conference in Las Vegas (if you can't tell, I seem to have great epiphanies at these conferences), I stumbled upon a class called, "The Book in You." I was like, *really*? God replied, *Yes, really*. After another long lecture and many more pages of notes, I once again found a secluded area to have a snack and decompress for a few minutes. It was then that I decided to take the bull by the horns and reach out to the publisher. I was thinking, I am going to do this. Everything is lining up and God is directing my steps. The publisher was excited and so was I...until I got home and real life kicked in. For me, "real life" meant, where the heck was I going to find time to write a book? Sure, I could have used things I'd already written, but the truth was that I was not in the same place spiritually, mentally, or physically as I'd been back then. No, to do this properly and from a place of authenticity I would have to start from scratch. August flew by and September was nearing its conclusion when a church sermon by Pastor Scott entitled "God Sent his Spirit" spoke to me. Suddenly I realized that all these messages about writing a book affirmed that God was choosing me to be a lighthouse, to bear witness about His light. I could clearly see the task before me, and what I had to do to make it happen. As soon as I realized it was not about me and more about lighting the way for others, the once insurmountable task of writing this book became a blessing. It was all at once deeply humbling and deeply empowering.

There is no doubt in my mind that each of us has a purpose to shine God's light, in the authentic way He has specifically entrusted us with. He qualifies us in the spirit and urges us to have faith in the mind and body, giving us the opportunity to fulfill His purpose. This was why I struggled with the idea of writing a book—I was looking for qualification in the flesh and ignoring my spirit. The foundational truth is that we do not have to be qualified by a degree or any other piece of paper; we come here endowed with all the qualifications we need by our

Creator. God has sent me, just as He has sent you. He has appointed me to shine His light, just as He has appointed you. That said, it is not about me and it is not really about you either. It is about the many people we are destined to touch with His light and truth. We are always seeking validation, qualification, and admiration from others and if we do not get it, we believe we have failed and that all our efforts have been a waste. Truly I say to you, our biggest failure lies in not acknowledging ourselves as qualified lighthouses, sent by the most high God. If we rewire our belief from "we work for the man" to "we work for God" then we will be witnesses for Him by walking, acting, and reacting with light to the natural disappointments we face within ourselves and in life. More importantly, God picks people like you and me to experience life in the spirit-mind-body so that we can shine His light and share it with others. I often hear, "There is something so very different about you but I can't put my finger on it." Well, I can. Now I believe that I am qualified to serve in whatever capacity God presents me with. Sometimes that scares me, but once I pray, poop, (yes, I said poop; it is part of my process) and talk to my lifelines—I commit to going wherever He sends me. The good news is that you have this opportunity too, but it is up to you to own it! It definitely took me some time, but I finally received the message loud and clear. We are qualified for whatever He presents to us and this truth is a cornerstone to becoming divinely fit. Be a witness and commit to be the lighthouse keeper you were destined to be.

SPIRIT-MIND-BODY EXERCISE

SPIRIT: Whenever you need reassurance, recite the mantra, "I commit to walking in light" or pray, "Lord, I commit to bearing witness to Your light with every step I take."

MIND: Make a list of all the qualifications, certifications, and trainings you have under your belt. Now google the different ways in which God refers to us in the Holy Bible. Compare the lists and assess which is of more value when it comes to achieving true happiness, self-worth, and confidence.

BODY: Do 25 jumping jacks as you recite the above mantra or prayer. Repeat as needed.

The Promise of Prayers

Do not be anxious about anything, but in everything, by prayer
and petition, with thanksgiving, present your requests to God.
And the peace of God, which transcends all understanding,
will guard your hearts and your minds in Christ Jesus.
Philippians 4:6-7

In the months leading up to my first wedding, I managed to shed eighty pounds. My job as a police officer had played a role in packing on the weight and in my decision to lose it. After being nearly dragged to my death while on the job, I began second-guessing myself, wondering whether I could have avoided the incident if I was in better shape. At that time, I was unaware that the external weight simply mirrored the internal weight I had been carrying around for many years; I was just happy to be a slim bride! I kept if off for the first couple of years of my marriage, even when I became pregnant. Then, when I hit my eighth month, I became very ill and ballooned right back to being eighty pounds overweight. Right now, you're probably thinking this is understandable, considering the circumstances. I simply considered it a failure. Regardless of the reason, the weight gain brought back all of my childhood baggage and feelings of insecurity, feelings that were only exacerbated by the discovery of my husband's infidelity. These stresses, coupled with the responsibilities of caring for my new daughter and a case of post-partum depression, proved overwhelming. It was time to make decisions about my marriage and about my life. Life didn't stop for my crisis.

Before I knew it, it was time to go back to work with this extra weight on. It was time to tuck in my shirt so I could carry my gun properly as a plainclothes detective. And, it was time to go and stand in front of over fifty people and lead an exercise class. What! My negative body image took over my mind and became the focus of each day. I felt like I had reached for God and He wasn't there. "Don't you know that I have a reputation to live up to?" I pleaded with Him, "Why are You doing this to me?!"

I remember standing in front of a large mirror, overcome with anxiety as I gasped at my reflection. For what stared back at me was appalling. A month after giving birth I was still wearing maternity underwear, and oh, my skin! I began pulling on the skin hanging from my abdomen and becoming more and more frantic as I realized that the loose flesh nearly reached my thighs. It was also darker than on the rest of my body and had the appearance and texture of elephant skin. My anxiety grew stronger and stronger by the second. It got so bad that I began to correlate the hanging skin with the many things in my life I wish I could change but couldn't. I thought, if only I could take a knife and cut off that hanging skin, all the abuse, neglect, loneliness, fear, helplessness, and depression would be gone as well. I was creating a story in my head that this would make everything okay.

It was then that the room darkened, and I dropped to my knees, exhausted. Then, suddenly, I felt a ray of light come from deep within my spirit. I immediately called out to God and asked for forgiveness. Forgiveness for being so vain, because at the root of my desperation and anxiety was the fact that I deeply cared about what people thought of me. I asked for forgiveness that I let my mind and body control my spirit by feeding it with lies. That day and night, I prayed on my hands and knees as I sobbed uncontrollably. I begged God for the faith to fuel my personal motivation, inspiration, strength, courage, and love for myself. I even asked Him to fill me with the confidence to believe that I have the privilege of giving Him my anxiety. In that moment, I realized that my mind is only clear when I let go of the need to look a certain way or to be accepted and instead look to God.

Have you experienced this kind of desperation and anxiety? If so, you know it applies not only to your physical appearance, but to every facet of your life. Living up to other people's expectations, be it your kids, coworkers, significant others, or even strangers, can push you so hard that your mind and body create a negative space for you to dwell in. This negativity lives between your ears and sabotages your efforts to workout, eat healthy, achieve goals, seek success, and take healthy risks. But if you give your anxiety to God, He will give you peace over your spirit, so it can guard your mind, heart, and body. Building a relationship with God through prayer is the key to your spiritual strength and life's success. Start small, and you will soon see His hand at work. Before you know it, you will be praying to Him about all the things you can and cannot change. I still struggle occasionally with what people think (I am human, after all!), but thanks to my daily prayers and petitions, the time I spend doing this has gone from 100% to 10%. I schedule prayer time in the mornings and if that doesn't work out I pray in the car, while waiting for a client, or at night when I finally nestle into bed. I have even incorporated "active prayer" into my life, meaning I pray right when something is going on. This allows me to stay "prayed up" in the face of any negativity and prevents me from saying or doing something I am sure

> *Building a relationship with God through prayer is key to your spiritual strength and life's success.*

to regret later. You can recite a prayer found on the internet or have an old-fashioned conversation with God—there is no right or wrong way to do it. Remember, God has been on your team since you were formed in your mother's womb; to become divinely fit you need only usher Him into all areas of your life through prayers and intercessions.

SPIRIT-MIND-BODY EXERCISE

SPIRIT: If you encounter a situation that causes you immediate anxiety, take 4 deep breaths, holding them in for a count of 4, then exhaling for a count of 4. Recite the mantra, "I will have peace over the things I cannot change" or pray for God's grace to cover you and His peace to fill you. Say, "May the Peace of God cover (fill in the area(s) of your life creating the anxiety)."

MIND: Make a list of the top 5 things that cause you anxiety. Circle the things you have control over and "X" the things you do not; this will give you new perspective. As you begin to pray on these things, make sure to journal about the changes you see; this will increase your trust in the spirit to lead your mind and body. Note: Be sure to schedule prayer time, even if it's only 5 minutes a day.

BODY: While reciting the mantra or prayer, do a series of 15 Downward-Facing Dogs to plank holds. This will release the feel-good hormones in your body and create a peaceful state.

The Promise of Rest

Come to Me, all you who are weary and burdened,
and I will give you rest.
Matthew 11:28

I grew up poorer than most of my peers at church school and summer camp, and though I didn't realize it at the time, being around them made me feel depressed. I vividly remember hearing their stories about ski vacations, what they received for birthdays and holidays, and how they thought learning to drive in a Mercedes was perfectly normal. They also looked perfect—at least I thought they did—with golden locks, beautiful light eyes, flawless white skin, and all the right clothes to fit their perfect bodies. I didn't resent them, exactly; I was too busy being down about my caramel-colored skin that got ashy, hair that got frizzy, a frame that was not a size zero, and clothes that were hand-me-downs or just not of the same caliber as those worn by my friends. I remember a feeling of helplessness, too, because these were things I could not change. Drawing these comparisons each Sunday and summer definitely stuck with me. Sometimes, it even knocked me down. I can remember borrowing their clothes and hoping they wouldn't ask for them back. At camp, when I went to chapel I prayed that my skin would turn lighter and my eye color would change; I bargained with God, promising to do this or that if He granted my wishes. Sometimes, I would lay on my bunk during rest hour and pray that all this would just go away. Obviously, these wishes weren't granted, because they were ridiculous and unrealistic; I would have to figure out how to release this burden to my spirit. This lesson took years to learn, but when I did, I felt renewed and refreshed; I even came to realize that I enjoyed every part of being different and what once depressed me now made me happy. I allowed the burden of circumstance and the cause of my depression to rest in God.

We need only look around to see that no one is free of burdens; everyone has things in their life that, if they allow it, can cause despair and weariness. For example, one person is depressed because they crave space from their spouse, while another is depressed because they do not have someone with whom to share their space. One person is depressed because they cannot lose the last ten pounds to reach their ideal weight and another is depressed about having to lose one hundred fifty pounds before they can have a

> *Calling upon your spirit to carry your burdens won't immediately solve the problem, but it will create space for you to rest, stop the spinning of your wheels, and receive God's peace and tranquility.*

mandatory surgery. One is depressed because their twenty-five-year-old son is a drug addict, and another is depressed because their child decided not to go to college. One is depressed because she has stretchmarks from her pregnancy while another is depressed because she cannot have children. One is depressed because she can't afford a tummy tuck while another is depressed because she looks worse after having one. One is depressed because he can't find a job while another is depressed because he doesn't like the job he has. One is depressed because he can't afford his dream car while another is depressed because he cannot afford *any* car. By no means does one cancel out or minimize the other—the point here is to gain perspective in the spirit when your mind tries to tell you that you are alone or that your problems are worse than everyone else's.

Burdens are life circumstances you are helpless over. Burdens weigh on the mind and cause depression, addictions, and bad habits. They wreak havoc on your relationships with others and steal your joy. They rob you of spiritual, mental, and physical rest. That's when your spirit can step in. Calling upon your spirit to carry your burdens won't immediately solve the problem, but it will create space for you to rest, stop the spinning of your wheels, and receive God's peace and tranquility. Remember, what cannot be done in man, God will do. Still, you must do your part to release your burdens, especially the ones that do not belong to you. Really look at your situation and ask yourself, am I committed to depression or am I committed to releasing my burdens? Consciously or subconsciously, you will eventually commit to one or the other. The choice is yours and yours alone. I know it is hard because the struggle is real in everyone and everywhere. Rest your burdens in the spirit and give yourself permission to move forward.

SPIRIT-MIND-BODY EXERCISE

SPIRIT: When those burden-filled thoughts arise, recite this mantra, "I release my burdens" or the prayer, "God, please take my burdens."

MIND: What are the top 3 things that cause you to become depressed? Are you helpless in the face of these circumstances, or are there actions you can take to alleviate them? Once you've answered these questions, allow yourself to pace around the room and truly feel your circumstances. Feel free to cry and scream but give it a time limit. No more than one hour. If you chose to spend it in bed, set your alarm.

BODY: Get your bearings with deep breaths. Add 50 high knees as you recite the above mantra or prayer and you will get a natural buzz. You will also gain the clarity of realizing that no one has time to be depressed. Moving on!

The Promise of Spiritual Intercession

Likewise the Spirit helps us in our weakness.
For we do not know what to pray for as we ought,
but the Spirit himself intercedes for us with groanings too
deep for words. And he who searches hearts knows what is
the mind of the Spirit, because the Spirit intercedes
for the saints according to the will of God.
Romans 8:26-27

I have seen the Spirit work in many ways to ease pain or simply carry us through life-altering situations. As a young adult I watched a woman of faith pray every minute of the day for her son to stay out of trouble. Not even a year after the trouble started, her son was shot and bled to death on a city street. As a mother, I cannot even fathom how difficult it must be to lose a child, but I saw this woman's light dim before my very eyes. At times she seemed to barely breathe because it hurt to do so. It was as if her sorrow had consumed her—spirit, mind, and body. Some time passed, and when I saw her again I noticed that something about her was different. She was still grieving her son's death, but she had come back to life. Amazed by what I was seeing, I asked her what had changed. She told me that her pain had been unbearable, and that she had been overwhelmed with helplessness, both when her son was alive and after he died. Her only comfort was God. He filled her spirit with love and allowed her weakness to become her strength. She told me God had interceded with her pain and gave her the same peace her son experienced when he passed away. There is no scientific explanation for this shift, only *the truth:* the spirit intercedes according to our willingness and the ultimate will of God. This woman is living testimony and I witnessed it.

I too have struggled with feelings of helplessness, especially when it comes to my kids. When I married my current husband, we merged families like the Brady Bunch—well, not quite. He came to the relationship with two boys—one, a quiet teen and the other, a tough preteen; I came in with my school age daughter, who fell somewhere in between. These young people would be the deliverers of some of my greatest lessons. See, I had dedicated my life to helping others, and over the years I'd inspired thousands, in word and in deed, in person and virtually, so it was difficult to accept that I might not always be able to reach or inspire the kids living under my own roof. It was scary for me to see them accepting mediocrity and living closer to today's culture than to their God-given potential, and even scarier when they dismissed my concerns. Their daily choices, actions, and reactions overwhelmed me with a feeling of helplessness. In this regard I am no different than most parents: our children are our greatest weakness and present the greatest challenges to our spirits, minds, and bodies. However, as I mentioned before, they are also our greatest teachers. When fights broke out between me and my daughter, I quickly learned that screaming at the top of my lungs or smacking her didn't resolve anything; in

> *You must choose to rest in the spirit and allow God to bring you the peace only He can bring.*

fact, it sometimes left me feeling even more helpless (other than the times she needed a good whack)! I now understand that this behavior was less about her than it was about my failure to trust God; I was trying to control the situation, instead of allowing Him to intercede for me in my time of weakness. I knew it was time to let Him out of the box and into all areas of my life. This goes for any problem—remember, nothing is too large, or too small, for God to handle.

I know this may sound farfetched because as a parent, it is never easy to get a call from a hospital nurse, teacher, another parent, police officer, or court official complaining of your child's behavior, just as it's not easy to hear your child in distress. In that moment we ask ourselves, who taught him/her to act that way? Where did he/she learn that from? And, our natural, yet defensive, response is, "I have done my best to guide him/her, where did I fail?" Well, you didn't. Like every other person on the planet, our children have personal choice, the free will given to us by God. Where we do fail our children is by not holding them accountable for their actions. It gives them a built-in excuse to do what they "want" to do versus what they "have" to do. In letting them off the hook we also contribute to their feeling of helplessness, as well as our own. Remember, for the most part children mirror the behaviors they see in their parents. The best we can do for those we love is give them an example of a spirit-led life; this will instill in them an internal peace that for the most part will keep them grounded through life's inevitable ups and downs.

That said, there are parents out there who do not set a good example for their children; they may even set an example of neglect or abuse. The good news is that no matter what we learned to mirror while growing up, we always have the power to change our reflection. Look at it this way: if you were to look in the mirror and see that your lips are chapped, you could adjust the reflection by taking action (i.e. applying Chapstick). This is a simple example, but the same ideology applies to every area of your life. That means it also applies to your children. They are capable of self-reflection and self-initiated change and should be held accountable to such. Your peace of mind and body cannot depend upon their choices. You must choose to rest in the spirit and allow God to bring you the peace only He can bring. Why should we confront issues alone when we can let God intercede for us?

I can distinctly remember various points in my life when I decided to relinquish my feelings of helplessness to God and felt an inexplicable peace. I have also witnessed others go through the same process. Yes, in some cases, this request for intercession occurred only after I tried utilizing several different tactics to resolve an issue and realized that I couldn't handle or control it, but that's okay, because at least I finally realized it! What can you really do when they call and tell you that you have cervical cancer? That you have Stage 4 breast cancer? That your child will only live to the age of sixteen? That you are being laid off? That your home has been swept away by a hurricane? That your husband lost his life at a concert he went to last night or that your sister was killed in a drive-by shooting? Wake up! You cannot control any of this. All you can do is pray for the Lord to intercede because in the flesh we are weak but in the spirit we are strong. His intercession can help you be strong enough to get you up in the morning, to keep you moving throughout the day and even get you to a workout. Yes, a workout! Personally, I always use my workouts to help awaken my spirit. I believe that a workout grounded in the spirit can be used as a template for life. A workout requires a person to schedule the time and kind of workout, get the proper clothing together, ensure their household responsibilities are taken care of, eat properly and drink enough water for fuel throughout the day, get to a workout facility, start the workout with faith, get through the workout with power, end the workout with energy, and do it all over again the next day. Sounds like the cycle of life to me. Do you agree? When we allow our feelings of helplessness to rest in God, He will empower the spirit, ease the mind, and give the body peace and rest, in all areas of life.

SPIRIT-MIND-BODY EXERCISE

SPIRIT: Recite this mantra, "My spirit trumps my mind and body," and/or pray over the things you will list below as sources of helplessness. Ask for God to intercede on your behalf and when your mind wanders and your body fails you, recite this short prayer, "Spirit, fill me in my weakness."

MIND: Name 5 things that are creating feelings of helplessness in your life right now. Circle the things you can change and "X" the things you cannot. Pray for clarity with regard to the steps you should take for all the things you circled. For the things you have X'd, see the spirit exercise above and pray for God's intercession.

BODY: Add 100 forward arm circles (arms out to your side at shoulder level) to feel strong and confident as you recite the mantra or prayer.

The Promise of the Supernatural

I can do all things through Him who strengthens me.
Philippians 4:13 ESV

If you're on social media, you've probably noticed that a lot of people love to post the above verse. I'm not knocking them for it—in fact, I applaud anyone who has the courage in this day and age to profess Christ. That said, it's one thing to "like," "share", and "tweet" something and another to apply it wholeheartedly to your life. You might say (or think) in the middle of an argument, "Lord give me strength," but do you really believe it? You can say, "Jesus, take the wheel" while dealing with a difficult person or situation, but do you *know* He will? Like a child with a parent, most of us tend to call upon Him only when we are in trouble, but what about when things are going well? We must remember that Christ not only strengthens us in our times of need, but He helps us live each day free from anxiety, if we choose to trust Him. Just to be clear, we will all have to endure suffering, but we must learn to shift the focus from our limited strength to His everlasting strength. I know this, because for years I tried doing things on my own and it didn't quite work out for me.

Though it was many years ago, I can vividly remember watching helplessly as my one-year-old daughter spiked yet another high fever. These fevers, which ranged from 102 to 104 degrees, had remained a mystery to her doctor, and not knowing what else to do I had been alternating between Tylenol and Motrin, along with her antibiotics, to keep them in check. But this was of course just masking the problem, and one day I'd had enough. I decided to take her to the emergency room and stay there until I got answers. And that's exactly what happened...sort of. My daughter was admitted for an unknown infection and kept in the hospital for five days. I was able to hold it together until they inserted a catheter inside her, and then I broke down—something I rarely did. My mother was there, and I remember looking at her and knowing she was in active prayer. I put my head down and did the same, saying "I can do all things through Christ who strengthens me," over and over. I was relentless. And although my daughter's condition was touch and go, I started to feel an incredible peace blanketing me, which in turn allowed me to comfort her. Through Christ, I had the strength to handle what I was not able to do alone.

The point I am making is that we often wait until we are truly desperate before calling on the spirit. In the flesh we believe we are strong enough and tough enough to do it on our own, only to "order" God to take over when we decide to quit. We forget that we can call on Him anytime, not just when things get dire. He always has been and always will be our supernatural superhero, ready to intercede. We need only to get out of our mind, hand the reins to our spirit, and walk with confidence that He is in control. The next time you post the verse on social media or on your phone's wallpaper, ask yourself whether you are daring to apply it to your life. Remember, when you depend on what you see or hear in the flesh, you are short-circuiting your access to God's supernatural powers. Now, who in their right mind would knowingly do that? Hopefully, not you!

We have all witnessed people with seemingly insurmountable struggles and asked ourselves, how does he or she do it? Take the mother who is caring around the clock for her mentally handicapped son. In the natural, she would not be able to do this for very long; it is too exhausting. Yet somehow, she goes on. Or how about the single parent who manages to juggle kids, a job (or two), and a million other things? They do it by making a choice each day to scrap by in the flesh or sustain it in the spirit. When we live in our minds and bodies, we get overwhelmed, exhausted and "stuck." This is when we are likely to stay in bed, drink alcohol, eat excessively or not eat at all, use drugs, cheat, hurt others, and engage in a whole host of other self-destructive behaviors. But when we recognize and truly believe that we can do all things through Christ, God's strength will begin to manifest in unimaginable ways. Now, this doesn't necessarily mean that we will get what we want, as it may be different from God's plan for our lives, but know this: God plans to bless you abundantly

> But when we recognize and truly believe that we can do all things through Christ, God's strength will begin to manifest in unimaginable ways.

in those areas you have expressed faith in. Take refuge in this truth and hold onto your hats, because you're in for the kind of adventure only your supernatural superhero can deliver!

Also remember that God prepares His warriors. Ephesians 6:14-18 reminds us to "Stand firm then, with the belt of truth buckled around your waist, with the breastplate of righteousness in place, and with your feet fitted with the readiness that comes from the gospel of peace. In addition to all this, take up the shield of faith, with which you can extinguish all the flaming arrows of the evil one. Take the helmet of salvation and the sword of the Spirit, which is the word of God. And pray in the Spirit…" Making a choice to wear the armor of God will deliver the transparency we all consciously and subconsciously seek in our lives.

So, stand firm. This doesn't mean one leg in and one leg out. It means both feet are planted, knees slightly bent, shoulders back so you can lead with your heart, just as if you were preparing to engage in a power squat or face an opponent in a fight. It means the belt of His truth is wrapped around the waist, securing the breastplate that can deflect all things. With your feet grounded in God's peace, holding up the shield of faith and wearing the helmet of salvation, you will be a warrior in God's army. With a supernatural superhero on your team, no weapon formed against you shall prosper, as written in Isaiah 54:17.

SPIRIT-MIND-BODY EXERCISE

SPIRIT: Whenever you need extra strength, recite the mantra, "I just have to be 1% stronger" or the prayer, "Jesus, take the reins." Record in a journal or on your phone the number of times you are triumphant in one day. This will be your motivation for the days that follow.

MIND: List 4 areas in your life in which you can use God's supernatural strength (i.e. time management or saving money). Write these 4 things on a sticky note and place it on a mirror in your home, your computer at work, or someplace else you'll be sure to see it on a regular basis. When dealing with time management issues, I wrote "God, help me not be late" on my sticky note. Every time I saw it, I was reminded that I didn't have to cram that "one more thing" into my day and that He would give me the strength to get it done. Try it!

BODY: While reciting the above mantra or prayer, do full sit-ups until you feel confident over the area(s) of your life in which you feel weak. The up-and-down motion of the exercise symbolizes the struggle, as well as the opportunity to show our strength and get back up.

The Promise of Spirit

Not only so, but we also glory in our sufferings, because we know that suffering produces perseverance; perseverance, character; and character, hope. And hope does not put us to shame, because God's love has been poured out into our hearts through the Holy Spirit, who has been given to us.
Romans 5:3

I have experienced and survived sexism, racism, classism, and probably a lot of other "isms" than I care to remember. My first marriage ended in divorce, but I am now blessed with a happy marriage and a beautiful daughter and sons. I had cervical cancer and I no longer do. I could've been a statistic, but I am not. I guess what I am trying to say is, yes, I have suffered but not nearly as much as others. Furthermore, those challenging experiences have made me who I am today.

Every single hardship in my life, every experience in this book (good or bad) has built my character. This growth and change happened organically, through my spiritual walk. See, God never promised the followers of Christ wouldn't go through any trials or tribulations. In fact, He assures us that we will continue to face the enemy and his evil ways, not to hurt us, but to test our faith and mold us. With every tribulation we will build perseverance and, if we lean on Him, we will find hope. Depending on what we are facing, we can call on this hope to get us through each second, minute, hour, day, month, year, and decade, until we are called to heaven. Yes, it can be very difficult—even unrealistic—to glorify God in the midst of hardship but it can be done.

The day I was told I had cervical cancer, the nurse put her hand on mine and asked, "How are you doing with the news? I would be a mess."

Imagine her shock when I just looked at her and replied, "It could be so much worse." I meant it, too. In fact, I don't believe I cried once. I had no chemo, no pills, just two procedures with no harsh side effects or significant down time. I believe this had something to do with my decision to strive in every situation. I know I cannot do that without being spirit-driven. What does this mean? It means I understand that Jesus died for my sins and God has through His sacrifice forgiven us all for our iniquities and allowed us to live in a judgement-free zone. He has freed us from bondage and given us an authentic temple to live in. He offers us daily balance through prayers and intercessions. He offers to be our living water as an alternative to living for the ways of the world. He promises to provide us with armor, insurance, and rest. He builds up our character through every experience and tribulation. In turn it is our choice to glorify Him by living with hope. We are "sent people," meaning God has sent us into the world to spread His light and His truth. If we lead a life that builds a transparent relationship among our spirit-mind-body, that will ensure the checks and balances and we need to become and remain divinely fit.

> *I believe this had something to do with my decision to strive in every situation. I know I cannot do that without being spirit-driven.*

SPIRIT-MIND-BODY EXERCISE

Below I have included the final spirit-mind-body exercise. As you do it, rejoice in the fact that you now have the tools to own living in the spirit and to lead in the Divinely Fit movement!

SPIRIT: Recite the mantra, "My struggle will ignite my perseverance," or the prayer "God, be my strength as I walk into my destiny of perseverance."

MIND: Write down at least two items for each of these: Times you have been forgiven for iniquities; provided a judgement free zone; shielded and/or freed from the bondage of a bad situation; healed from an illness or injury; had your prayers answered; intercessions made; provided assurance or rest. Writing this down will make you see that God has always been with you and is using this book as a vessel to make you aware of that fact and His undying love for you.

BODY: Search on your phone for Chris Tomlin's "God's Great Dance Floor" or any other Christian or gospel song that resonates with you. Blast it and have a party with your spirit. Dance the whole song, listen to the words, and let it rejuvenate you and fill you with the confidence of the spirit you will now use to lead your life!

My Divinely Fit Wish for You

It is my wish that you use this book as a tool on your life's journey. Open it when you feel challenged. Read it when you need inspiration or encouragement. Share the lessons with a friend who is going through a hard time. Allow my life to be a reflection for your own. Know that if I can make it through my struggles by calling on God's promises to empower your spirit, you can too. Commit to struggling with your dark roots in the divine spirit, and God's promises will illuminate all the areas of your life.

You are a warrior and a child of God. You are equipped and worthy. May you feel His blessing every day of your life and may you embrace the power of being DIVINELY FIT, spirit. mind, and body.

Massive Love and Namaste`
Karla

Acknowledgements

First, I would like to offer a very special thanks to those who taught me early on that I would never live up to others' expectations—you inspired me to work not only harder but smarter, and to turn to God to help me overcome and achieve what I never could have done alone.

Funny, I almost did not write an acknowledgements section. I figured my friends and family already know how much I value them. But then I remembered that you should never let an opportunity to say *thank you* or *I love you* pass by.

To my core group of family and friends, you are amazing teachers and supporters and I love you from the depths of my soul. To my mom, thanks for giving me life and blessing me with my Taino roots. To my biggest sis, thanks for always seeing me. To my big sis, you are my hero for doing all that you do—not only for me but for so many—thank you. To other siblings, my children, and my nephews and nieces, leaving a legacy to you is what keeps me chasing who I want to be in five years. To my daughter, Jules my peanut, thank you for showing me how to open my heart and setting the foundation for me to love and be loved. To my husband, you are the one that always says, "You can do that!"—no matter what it is—thank you for your unwavering support and for always being my rock.

To my Sudor Taino team and tribe, thanks for your support and motivating me to be the best every single day. Some of you have been with me since the beginning and some of you promote everything I do, and that means everything to me!

To my mentors, acquaintances, and spiritual mentees, thank you for accepting yesterday's me, today's me, and the me I will be in the future. Thanks to my pastor (WEFC), his wife, and my community group for giving me weekly spiritual direction and inspiration, and to my accountability partner for your tireless tenacity, business expertise, and no-nonsense approach to handling me and life!

I also want to thank the countless other teachers I have encountered in my life. I believe that every person, from the janitor and prisoners I met during my booking assignment to my rockstar sister-cousins play distinct roles in my journey to spiritual freedom.

Everyone has had a hand in pointing me in the right direction: GFF (God Family and Fitness on all levels—spiritual, mental, and physical).

About Sudor Taino®
Group Fitness Studio

Sudor Taino serves people of all shapes and sizes with an innovative training philosophy and the ideology of breathing fitness & life with passion. Karla founded this studio on the principal of finding what moves people in an effort to better humankind.

SPECIAL OFFER - EXPERIENCE SUDOR TAINO!

Contact us today to receive a free week of unlimited and innovative classes (newcomers only), free consultations, or 20% off any pass, membership, customized training, guided stretch, or nutritional service. On Facebook, be sure to like our page and sign up for our free online challenge group!

Sudor Taino Group Fitness
635 New Park Avenue
West Hartford CT. 06111
860-952-9015

About the Author

Karla C. Medina
Entrepreneur, Master Trainer, Author

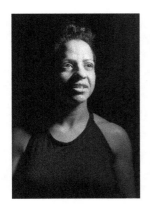

Karla is a passionate, Latina entrepreneur and renowned fitness guru who is highly respected for her no-nonsense innovative approach to business and life. She holds many local and national press, book publication and video production credits.

Karla is also a 20-year retired Police Sergeant veteran of the Hartford Police Department and is currently a State of Connecticut Training Officer. She has her B.S. in Business Management and master's degree in Public Policy along with many other certifications and trainings.

She is the owner and master trainer at Sudor Taino® Group Fitness, a studio dedicated to enhancing people's individual journey towards health, fitness, and life. Her spirit, mind, body approach contributes to her authentic style and allows her to move people individually, motivate them collectively, and move them culturally. Karla is known for being an energetic motivational speaker and heartfelt philanthropist. She promises to pursue her God given purpose.

Karla C. Medina
sudortaino@live.com
sudortaino.com
facebook.com/SudorTainoGroupFitness
IG: Sudor Taino Group Fitness Studio

Are You Called to be an Author?

Join the Wisdom & Insights Series of Inspirational Teaching Guides.

If you're like most people, you may find the prospect of writing a book daunting. Where to begin? How to proceed? No worries! We're here to help.

The book you're holding is part of our Wisdom & Insights Series. We've created this series to deliver lessons, stories, and practices to assist individuals in various aspects of spiritual development and personal growth. As an author, you'll use our QuickPublish Formula™ designed to help you to write your book with ease.

Whether you choose to be part of our Wisdom & Insights book series, write your own book, or contribute to an anthology, Powerful You! will be your guiding light, professional consultant, and enthusiastic supporter. If you see yourself as an author collaborating with a publishing company who has your best interest at heart and with the expertise to back it up, we're the publisher for you.

We provide personalized guidance through the writing and editing process. We offer complete publishing packages and our service is designed for a personal and optimal authoring experience.

We are committed to helping individuals express their voices and shine their lights into the world. Are you ready to start your journey as an author? Do it with Powerful You! Publishing.

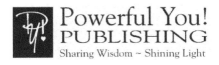

Powerful You! Publishing
239-280-0111
powerfulyoupublishing.com

9 780997 066180